MEDITERRA

COOKBOOK 2021

MOUTH-WATERING RECIPES TO KICK-START YOUR HEALTH GOALS

CATHERINE MOORE

DISCLAIMER

The information contained in the Book is for informational purposes only, and in no case may it constitute the formulation of a diagnosis or the prescription of treatment.
The information contained in the Book is not intended and should not in any way replace the direct doctor-patient relationship or the specialist visit.
It is recommended to always seek the advice of your doctor and/or specialists regarding any indication reported.

CONTENTS

CONTENTS

INTRODUCTION

Mediterranean diet is basically the diet of nations living on the Mediterranean Sea. The diet aims to increase the intake of healthy fats, fruits, and vegetables and decrease the intake of saturated fats, red meat, sugar and sodium. It emphasizes an increased intake of whole grains, nuts, seeds, and legumes.

WHAT IS MEDITERRANEAN DIET?

First of all, it is important to know that classic Mediterranean diet isn't just food, but rather, it is way of life.

Mediterranean diet is based on simplicity and frugality. The main goal is to prepare food as close to natural state, as possible.

Mediterranean diet is more about lifestyle than diet. The main features are balanced nutrition, with lots of fresh fruits, vegetables, fish, olive oil, vegetable oils with low levels of animal fats, moderate consumption of wine (preferably red) with meals, and active lifestyle, in all aspects of life. Mediterranean diet is also known for its low glycemic index, low nutritional density, low consumption of saturated fat, and low consumption of cholesterol. It is also very high in antioxidant and low in omega-6 fatty acids cholesterol. Studies have shown Mediterranean diet is highly protective against cancer, cardiovascular disease and diabetes. It's also known for its beneficial effects on the microbiome. Mediterranean diet has been shown to improve certain aspects of health: physical, mental and emotional. There is strong evidence that Mediterranean diet affects hormones, inflammatory response, microbiome and endocrine system.

It can be harmful if is eaten in wrong quantities, consumed at inappropriate times or eaten for too many years

What to Eat?

Regarding dietary necessities, such as specific component, we can clarify that:

Mediterranean plant-based diet: adequate intake of plant foods, vegetables, fruit, cereal grain, legume and extra-virgin olive oil.

Mediterranean animal-based diet: adequate intake of species with the lightest fats (poultry especially the dark meat, and egg), grapes, grapes and other berries, seeds and nuts, wine, vegetables (especially the green leafy ones), some vegetables and fruits (like olives and varieties of grapes).

Mediterranean fish-based diet: sufficient intake of species with the lightest fats (fish, shellfish), pasta, olive oil and other foods to increase intake of fat-soluble vitamins K, A and D, vegetables and fruits.

Should we go on and mention that although Mediterranean diet is quite diverse, the diet is healthy, but not balanced. This of course, means that a lean person should not focus on the ratio of protein and carbohydrates (like a person with diabetes would usually do) but on the quality of what he or she is eating. Mediterranean Diet, in the future (with more research and clinical studies) will be a paradigmatic example of healthy diet, with biological replicates which can be implemented in the western world. It's all about right balance with the right quantity of nutrients, the right quality, and the right time.

History of Mediterranean Diet

The Mediterranean diet is food patterns typical of the Mediterranean Basin, including southern Europe, northern Africa and Latin America. The origins of Mediterranean diet started with a study conducted by Ancel Keys in the 1970s, when he demonstrated that countries around the Mediterranean Sea had lower rates of cardiovascular disease than other parts of Europe. Thereafter, the Mediterranean diet was often connected with the lower rates of cardiovascular disease and cancer. Mediterranean diet is rich in fruits and vegetables, whole grains, legumes, nuts, and beans, as well as high in seafood, olive oil, and moderate in alcohol.

Benefits of the Mediterranean Diet

Here are the Benefits of the Mediterranean Diet:

This diet is known as perhaps the only one that provides you with good health in the long run. You will never feel hungry, nor will you feel as if though you are preventing yourself from eating delicious foods.

The only thing this diet requires is to reduce the consumption of unhealthy foods such as red meat, junk food, processed food, and sugars.

Mediterranean diet puts an accent on vegetables, fruits, seeds, fish, and legumes. You do not need to be a nutritionist or a doctor to know that a diet rich in such foods is a sure way to provide your body with healthy nutrients.

This diet is an extremely popular option for weight loss, but even if you are not willing to slim, you can switch to this diet because of the many health benefits it provides.

People who have heart and cardiovascular issues, skin problems, diabetes, or simply want to stay healthy and lower the risk of evil diseases (like cancer), are advised to start the Mediterranean diet.

Let's take a look at the health benefits that this diet brings.

Reduced Risk of Heart Failures

Providing your body with colorful meals that contain large amounts of fruits, vegetables, healthy oils, and lesser processed food or unhealthy ingredients is a sure way to remain in good health.

New England Journal of Medicine published a study in 2013 that was following more than 7000 people (men and women) in Spain who were suffering from type 2 diabetes. They were at high risk for cardiovascular illnesses; the ones that were following the Mediterranean diet (plenty of vegetables, fruits, fish, and olive oil) had about a 30% lower risk of heart failures. The researchers did not encourage the participants to exercise (the study wanted to see only the results of the diet).

The study reanalyzed the data in 2018, and they came with similar results.

Consuming large amounts of fish instead of red meat is the key to a healthy heart; the risk for seizures, heart attacks, cholesterol, and early death is reduced.

Prevents Alzheimer's Disease and Memory Decline

The Mediterranean way of eating will help your brain stay in good shape. As we get older, our memory tends to decline, and the brain's activity significantly drops.

The human brain needs food to function properly, and when that food is not suitable, the risk of diseases such as Alzheimer's grows higher.

Our brains need quality nutrients and oxygen, and the best way to provide that is by the right foods.

Food that is not providing our blood with enough oxygen will manifest in poor memory and cognitive functioning.

In 2016 the Journal Frontiers in Nutrition was monitoring the effect of the Mediterranean diet on the cognitive functions. The results showed that this diet does improve brain functioning and slows down memory declining.

Weight Loss and Healthy Weight Maintenance

Switching from a regular (mostly unhealthy) diet to the Mediterranean pattern of eating is a very common thing. This way of eating is not a new thing, nor was it created by nutritionists.

This is a regular lifestyle of the people who live around the Mediterranean (Spain, France, Italy, Balkan countries).

The menu consists of foods that are native to the area, especially fruits, vegetables, seeds, fish, nuts, herbs.

What makes this eating pattern so suitable for weight loss is the fact that it suggests consuming fresh and whole-food without additional additives that only add flavor and make you crave more unhealthy foods. The purging effect of fruits, vegetables, nuts, and healthy fats like olive oils cleanses your body from fat and cholesterol and helps in the slimming process.

The body is now provided with healthy nutrients that are easy for digestion. Healthy fats (olive oil, avocado, nuts) provide the brain and the body with sufficient amounts of energy, while the rest of the ingredients are not layered in fats all over the body.

Consuming this calorie-unrestricted Mediterranean eating pattern for five years will keep your weight balanced.

The food combination in its suggested amounts (daily, weekly, and monthly) will result in a healthy weight loss.

If your goal is to lose a larger amount of weight, you can combine the Mediterranean diet with calorie restriction and physical activity.

Mediterranean Diet Helps in Managing Type 2 Diabetes

People who have type 2 diabetes are advised to follow diets that are not rich in carbohydrates and sugars. The Mediterranean diet might be a good solution for them, as well.

This diet is all about whole grains and healthy carbohydrates, which will not increase the blood sugar levels. Complex whole-grain carbohydrates (quinoa, wheat berries, or buckwheat) are a far better option than refined carbohydrates (white bread, sweets, juices, chocolate, fast food).

Studies show that people aged 50 to 80 years, who were diabetes-free and followed the Mediterranean diet for three to four years, did not develop the disease.

These people used olive oil and nuts, and in general, ate whole food and fish instead of processed food and meats. They had a 52% lower risk for type 2 diabetes.

Mediterranean Diet Reduces the Risk of Some Cancers

Food can be both cure and poison. When your daily menu contains foods rich in unhealthy fats (palm oil, butter), red meat, processed food, sugars, and large amounts of proteins (mostly from red meat) and carbohydrates (unhealthy options such as cookies, white bread, rice, French fries, etc.) – your body will suffer on the long run.

Most cancers are a result of poor eating habits, lack of physical activity, polluted air, and so on.

The Mediterranean diet helps in reducing the risk of cancers like colorectal, gastric, and breast cancer. The high intake of vegetables, fruits, and whole grains play a powerful role in keeping you healthy and in good shape.

Studies show that women who follow this diet (and use extra-virgin olive oil) have a 62% lower risk of breast cancer.

Mediterranean Diet Can Help with Anxiety and Depression

Almost everyone has experienced occasional depression (due to stress, problems in the family, or work).

Depression is a persistent loss of enthusiasm and enjoyment in doing things you once liked doing. Despair, lethargy, disinterest, sleeping problems are just a few of the symptoms of depression.

On the other hand, anxiety often manifests with nervousness before significant events, speaking to people, and meeting new people, going out, making mistakes, and fear of arguments. Sweaty palms, irritable bowel movement, overthinking, lack of sleep, and intrusive thoughts that you are not good enough or not doing things good enough are just a few of the symptoms.

Psychologists say that diet and mental health are tightly connected. Foods packed in healthy ingredients can seriously improve your general health, including your energy levels and mental state.

Suppose you avoid processed foods rich in unhealthy fats, red meat, white bread, and sugars. In that case, you will witness significant changes in every aspect of your life.

Change of the lifestyle (new eating habits and physical activity) can improve the depression and anxiety symptoms. Good, healthy, and quality food impacts the mood and increases the levels of serotonin. When physical activity is added, depression becomes less severe. Naturally, you need to see professional help from a therapist, but your diet change could only bring positive shifts.

This diet also affects the immune system, which is one of the main factors in the risk of depression.

When your body is at a high risk of inflammation, it is more prone to depression. According to the studies published in The Journal of Clinical Psychiatry, depressed people have a 46% higher risk of inflammatory diseases in their blood.

The Mediterranean diet is packed with anti-inflammatory foods – olive oil, leafy greens, nuts, salmon, sardines, oranges, strawberries are just some of the foods that fight inflammation.

On the other hand, foods like margarine, red meat, processed meat, deep-fried foods, white bread, soft drinks (soda and tetra pack juices) are not recommended because they are not healthy, but because they are known for their inflammatory properties.

TIPS TO START OFF

The healthy Mediterranean way of life is all about eating balanced foods rich in vitamins, minerals, antioxidants, and healthy fatty acids. However, the Mediterranean diet is just one aspect of it. The Mediterranean way of life calls for regular physical exercise, plenty of rest, healthy social interaction, and fun. Balancing all these aspects was the secret of the good health of the Mediterranean folk back in the day.

However, only the Mediterranean diet is the primary focus of this book. We will spend most of our time talking about just that.

Eat Healthy Fats

The Mediterranean diet is by no means a low-fat diet, but the fat included in this diet is considered healthy for the body, and the heart in particular. Remember: not all fats are created equal. Certain kinds of fats are healthy, while others do more harm than good. Monosaturated fats and polyunsaturated omega-3 fatty acids, for example, are considered healthy. Omega-6 polyunsaturated fatty acids and saturated fats are unhealthy.

These unhealthy fats are primarily present in most of the common food worldwide. The United States, for example, absolutely loves saturated fats. According to a survey, saturated fats constitute 11% of an average American's total calories, which is a very high number compared to an average Mediterranean resident, who consumes less than 8% of his/her calories through saturated fat.

If you wish to switch to the healthy Mediterranean way of life, the first thing to do is change the oils you consume.

Eliminating fats like butter and lard in favor of healthier oils like olive oil would be the place to start.

Consume Dairy in Moderation

We all love cheese. Dairy products are delicious, nutritious, and great sources of calcium. They should be consumed in moderation if you're following the Mediterranean diet.

It is usually a good idea to consume two to three servings of full-fat dairy products in a single day, where one serving can mean an 8-ounce glass of milk, or 8 ounces of yogurt, or an ounce of cheese.

Consume Tons of Plant-Based Foods

As we saw in the pyramid, fruits, vegetables, legumes, and whole grains form the basis of the Mediterranean diet. So, it is a good idea to eat five to ten servings of these in a single day, depending on your appetite. Eat as much of these as you want, but don't overeat. Plant-based foods are naturally low in calories and high in fiber and nutrients. Fresh unprocessed plants are best, so always be on the lookout for the best sources of these around you!

Spice Things Up with Fresh Herbs and Spices

Fresh herbs and spices make most of the recipes insanely delicious, while also providing health benefits. If you already use these in your daily cooking, more power to you! If not, we got you covered!

Consume Seafood Weekly

As we've talked before, one benefit of living close to the sea is easy to access to seafood. However, seafood holds a lower priority than plant-based foods in the Mediterranean diet and should be consumed in moderation. If you're a vegetarian, consider taking fish oil supplements to get those omega-3 fatty acids into your system.

Better yet, considering shunning your vegetarianism, and eating seafood to get the vital nourishment only seafood can provide.

Consume Meat Monthly

Red meat used to be a luxury for the Mediterranean people back in the day. Although not completely off-limits, you should try and reduce your red-meat intake as much as possible. If you love red meat, consider consuming it no more than two times per month. And even when you eat it, make sure the serving size of the meat in the dish is small (two to three-ounce serving). The main reason to limit meat intake is to limit the number of unhealthy fats going into your system.

As we talked before, saturated fats and omega-6 fatty acids are not good for health. Still, unfortunately, red meat contains significant quantities of these. As a beef lover myself, I eat a two-ounce serving of it per month, and when I do eat it, I make sure there are lots of vegetables on the side to satiate my hunger.

Drink Wine!

Love wine? Well, it is your lucky day. Having a glass of wine with dinner is a common practice in the Mediterranean regions.

Red wine is especially good for the heart and it is a good idea to consume a glass of red wine twice a week. Excess of everything is bad, and wine is no exception so keep it in check. Also, suppose you're already suffering from health conditions. In that case, it is a good idea to check with your doctor before introducing wine to your daily diet.

Work Your Body

Now you don't have to hit the gym like a maniac to work your body. Walking to your destination instead of driving, taking the stairs instead of the lift, or kneading your dough can all get the job done. So, be creative and work your body when you can. Better yet, play a sport or just hit the gym like a maniac. As I said at the start, you don't have to have to, but it will help... a lot.

Enjoy a Big Lunch

Lunch was usually the meal of the day when the Mediterranean residents sat with their families and took their time enjoying a big meal. This strengthens social bonds and relaxes the mind during the most stressful time of the day, when you're just halfway done with your work, probably.

Have Fun with Friends and Family

Just spending a few minutes per day doing something fun with your loved ones is great for de-stressing. Today, we don't understand the importance of this, and people feel lonely, and in some cases, even depressed.

Just doing this one thing has the power to solve a huge chunk of the problems our modern society faces.

Be Passionate

The Mediterranean people are passionate folk. Living on or close to sun-kissed coasts, their passion for life is naturally high. Being passionate about something in life can take you a long way towards health and wellness.

Planning Your Meals

Suppose you're a beginner and have not yet made the switch to the Mediterranean diet. In that case, you will need to identify what changes you need to make to your current diet to make it match closely with the Mediterranean diet.

In time, the Mediterranean diet will come to you naturally, but to start, you will need to plan. You will need to plan your portion sizes, and how often you eat certain foods. The changes are small but will benefit you in the long run.

Importance of Meal Planning

Meal planning is all about creating a road map for what you're going to eat, when you will prepare the food, and what ingredients you will need to buy. It might sound simple, but will save you from many headaches and make your transition to the Mediterranean diet much smoother. Meal planning is vital because:

- It enables you to be efficient with your time
- It enables you to plan what ingredients you will buy and when so that when you cook them, they are at their freshest
- You don't have to worry about what to cook multiple times per day. You take care of it in one sitting.
- It saves money by reducing food wastage. You cook everything you buy while it is still fresh.

Meal Planning Techniques

Meal planning is a flexible process, and every person has a unique way of going for it. You will eventually discover how you like to plan your meals, but it would be useful to look at a few templates of the common ways of doing it.

If you like to be moderately thorough and detailed, you can sit down and write what you will eat for breakfast, lunch, and dinner for each day of the week. If you like to munch on snacks from time to time, make sure you write those down too. Make sure the recipes you choose for that week are in season, and you can procure fresh ingredients for the written recipes.

• Suppose you like to get all the thinking for the whole month done in a single sitting. In that case, you can prepare meal plans for multiple weeks, along with shopping lists that specify what you will buy, and when, in such a way that the ingredients are at their freshest at the time of cooking. This will take a while, but a good place to start if you have the time. Just make sure you don't plan for too long, and make a new plan with every season to get the good seasonal stuff.

• Once you get slightly well acquainted with the diet, you will start to have the Mediterranean staples in your pantry at all times, and you don't need to plan all three meals per day or even your shopping list. You will have your favorite recipes that you will automatically shuffle as per your convenience. You will start to make larger batches so you can eat leftovers later if you're not in the mood to cook again. You might need to plan your big dinners once in a while, but that is about it.

In a nutshell, Mediterranean cooking will come to you naturally and will require minimal planning. Another great idea to keep in mind when you are on such a diet is to make a great shopping list. It will help you buy the right ingredients. Choose organic products if you can but only if they suit your budget. Your shopping list must include:

• Veggies like kale, garlic, spinach, arugula, onions, carrots

• Fruits like grapes, oranges, apples and bananas

• Berries like blueberries, strawberries, raspberries

• Frozen veggies

• Grains like whole-grain pasta, whole-grain breads

• Legumes like beans, lentils, chickpeas

• Nuts like walnuts, cashews, almonds

• Seeds like pumpkin seeds and sunflower seeds

• Condiments like turmeric, cinnamon, salt, pepper

- Shrimp and shellfish

- Fish like mackerel, trout, tuna, salmon and sardines

- Cheese
- Yogurt and Greek yogurt
- Potatoes and sweet potatoes
- Chicken

- Eggs
- Olives
- Olive oil and avocado oil

If you buy healthy and adequate ingredients, you will most certainly eat the right foods and you will definitely stay on your diet.

THE MEDITERRANEAN DIET PYRAMID AND SHOPPING LIST

— • • — ● — • • —

Mediterranean Diet Pyramid

The Mediterranean Diet Pyramid is a nutritional guide that was developed by the World Health Organization in 1993. It was also worked on by the Harvard School of Public Health, and the Oldways Preservation Trust. It is a visual tool that summarizes the Mediterranean Diet's suggested eating pattern and gives a guide to how frequently specific tools should be eaten. This allows you to break healthy eating habits and not overfill yourself with too many calories.

How is the pyramid laid out? Let's go over each tier.

Olive oil, fruits, vegetables, whole grains, legumes, beans, nuts & seeds, spices & herbs:

These are the types of food that form the Mediterranean pyramid base. You'll notice that these are mostly from plant sources. You should try and include a few variations of these items into each meal you eat. Olive oil should be the main fat you use in your cooking and your dishes, so replace any other butter or cooking oil you used to use. Generous uses of

herbs and spices are also encouraged

to season your food and add flavor as an alternative to salt. If you don't have access to fresh herbs, you can buy the dried version.

Always be sure to read the nutrition labels to ensure no other ingredients are mixed with the herbs. Fresh ginger and garlic are also great flavor enhancers for your meals. They can be easily stored in the freezer.

Fish & seafood: These are important staples of the Mediterranean diet that should be consumed often as a protein source. You want to try and include these in your diet at least two times a week.

Try new varieties of fish, either frozen or fresh. Also incorporate seafood like mussels, crab, and shrimp into your diet. Canned tuna is also great to include on sandwiches or toss in a salad with fresh vegetables.

Cheese, yogurt, eggs & poultry: These ingredients should be consumed in more moderate amounts when on the Mediterranean diet. Depending on the food, they should be used sparingly throughout the week. Remember that if you are using eggs in baking or cooking, those will also be counted in your weekly limit. You want to stick to more healthy cheese like Parmesan, ricotta, or feta that you can add as a topping or garnish on your dishes.

Red meat & sweets: These items will be consumed less frequently when on the Mediterranean diet. If you are eating them, you want to be sure it is only in small quantities and prefer lean meat versions with less fat. Most studies recommend a maximum of 12 to 16 ounces per month.

You can still have red meat on occasion to add some variety to your diet, but you want to reduce how often you have it. That's because of all the health concerns that come with sugar and red meat. The Mediterranean diet is working to improve cardiovascular health and reduce blood pressure, while red meat tends to be dangerous in cardiac health. Greece's residents ate very little red meat and instead had fish or seafood as their main source of protein.

Water: The Mediterranean diet encourages you to be hydrated, which means drinking more than your daily intake of water. The Institute of Medicine recommends a total of 9 cups each day for women, and 13 cups for men. If a woman is pregnant or breastfeeding, that number should be increased.

Wine: Moderate consumption of wine with meals is encouraged on the Mediterranean diet. Studies have shown that moderate consumption of alcohol can reduce the risk of heart disease. That can mean about 1 glass per day for women. Men tend to have higher body mass so they can consume 1 to 2 glasses. Please keep in mind what your doctor would recommend regarding wine consumption based on your health and family history.

Your Mediterranean Diet Shopping List

Includes:

Extra virgin and virgin olive oils: These will be the least processed and refined versions of olive oil on the market. They will contain the highest level of plant compounds called "phenols" that act as antioxidants in the body. It might be a little pricier than the oil you used before, but it's well worth it when you're aware of the health benefits you will gain! This will be your go-to when it comes to cooking, frying, seasoning, and as the base of your salad dressings. Remember, less is more!

Vegetables: You have pretty much free rein with vegetables though if you can stick to low-calorie ones, that's even better for your weight loss goals. Vegetables like zucchini, mushrooms, cabbage, cauliflower, bell pepper, and spinach are low in calories. However, they are still very filling and high in fiber. Try new vegetables and eat them in different ways like a green smoothie or different salad combinations to get bored. Try to buy in season items so you can save yourself some money!

Fruits: Fruits are encouraged and are great as a substitute healthy dessert to treat yourself to. Figs and pomegranates are native to the Mediterranean area, but any fruit will do! Be sure to include various colorful fruits and vegetables which allow you to have a diverse range of essential vitamins and minerals. If you have diabetes, try and consume fruits that are low on the glycemic index such as oranges, apples, grapefruits, pears, or plums.

Legumes & beans: These are a great hidden source of protein which often get overlooked in the West in favor of red meat or poultry items. Thankfully, the Mediterranean diet urges you to try different variations of protein sources! Whether it's black beans, kidney beans, chickpeas, or lentils, these are great to experiment with. Don't forget hummus! These are packed with fiber as well, so they allow you to feel full for longer. Be sure you drink plenty of water to avoid constipation!

Whole grain breads and cereal: Whether it's rice, barley, oats, leek rice, quinoa, whole grain pasta, or whole grain bread, you want to be sure you are focused on whole grains that are healthier rather than refined or processed grains. Same goes with cereal. Be sure you read the label and ensure the product is made from whole grain starches and are not processed into refined products. Ezekiel bread is a whole grain bread made with no sugar. One slice is packed with fiber and contains only 80 calories! The trick with whole grains is that you can eat a smaller portion than you would with refined wheat products but stay full longer. These are also low on the glycemic index scale which makes them safe for diabetes patients.

Nuts & seeds: This includes cashews, pistachios, walnuts, sunflower seeds, pine nuts, flax seeds, almonds, and other nuts which may be your favorites. Keep these as a healthy snack throughout the day but be sure to avoid the chocolate-covered or salted versions which are unhealthy. You want to stick to the raw nuts. Chia seeds are also tiny but powerful! In just 2 tablespoons, you can have 11 grams of fiber! These are great to add to a smoothie or topping on oatmeal or cereal to fill you up. The great thing is they're almost flavorless so anyone can incorporate them into their meals!

Low-fat dairy: If you are used to dairy products in your diet, you don't have to cut them out entirely but you should switch to low-fat versions. Use fat-free yogurt or low-fat cheese, and switch to skim or reduced fat milk. On the Mediterranean diet you want most of your dairy calories to come from healthy cheeses like feta, brie, Greek yogurt, or Parmesan.

Herbs & spices: These are great to season your food with and add a great distinct flavor other than salt. You can try using fresh herbs like rosemary and parsley though they may not last as long in your refrigerator. You can always start a windowsill herb garden which are easy to maintain! If not, don't be intimidated and feel free to use dried herbs from the spice aisle. Experiment with new flavors that will enhance your flavor profile. Fresh garlic and ginger are also great flavor enhancers and considered essentials of Greek and Mediterranean cuisine. They have multiple health benefits and pack your meals with flavor.

Excludes:

Red meat: As we mentioned, you want to go light on red meat portions when shopping for your Mediterranean diet. If you want to get a few pieces, be sure they're smaller sized and lean meat cuts with less fat. Try only to have it once a week and keep an eye on your portion size. Also, avoid high-fat processed meats like pre-made sausages or hot dogs loaded with preservatives and high in sodium. These tend to cause inflammation in the body.

Poultry:

Again, you want to use poultry in your diet less often than you would on other diets. More lean cuts with less fat can be used now and then as long as you have smaller portions. For the most part, try and substitute your red meat and poultry meals with fish or seafood, although it's okay to have them once in a while during the week. Turkey or duck would be a healthier alternative to chicken because they contain less fat.

Refined grains:

These include things like bagels, cereal, or white bread that we might previously consider staples in our diet. But these should be excluded from your shopping list unless you have verified that the cereals, pasta, or bread are whole grain certified products.

Sugars: That means skipping things like candy, chocolate, ice cream, sugary juices, and sodas! Instead, try and treat yourself to berries or fruit as a sweet treat, or enhance your water with lemon or mint leaves for more flavor. Get used to the habit of having natural sugars in fruit as a dessert instead of wanting unhealthy baked goods.

Trans or saturated fats: Exclude things like butter or margarine which contain unhealthy saturated fats. You want to substitute any unhealthy oils like canola oil or vegetable oil with the healthier option of extra virgin olive oil. You want to use this in your cooking, frying, and as your vinaigrettes' main component.

Highly processed foods: These should be avoided on the Mediterranean diet. The rule of thumb should be if it comes in a box, you can't have it! That's because food that tends to be marked as "low-fat" or "diet friendly" is very processed and unhealthy for you. Instead of eating those empty calories, focus on what you can eat as a filling snack like some of the items we mentioned above.

Pesto Dip

Prep Time: 5 min

Cooking Time: 0 min

Servings: 6

Ingredients:

- 1 cup cream cheese, soft 3 tablespoons basil pesto
- Salt and black pepper to the taste 1 cup heavy cream
- tablespoon chives, chopped

Directions:

1. In a bowl, mix the cream cheese with the pesto and the rest of the ingredients and whisk well.
2. Divide into small cups and serve as a party dip.

Nutrition:

calories 230, fat 14.5, fiber 4.8, carbs 6.5, protein 5.4

Feta Artichoke Dip

Prep Time: 10 min   **Cooking Time:** 30 min   **Servings:** 8

Ingredients:

- 8 ounces artichoke hearts, drained and quartered
- ¾ cup basil, chopped
- ¾ cup green olives, pitted and chopped 1 cup parmesan cheese, grated
- 5 ounces feta cheese, crumbled

Directions:

1. In your food processor, mix the artichokes with the basil and the rest of the ingredients, pulse well, and transfer to a baking dish.

2. Introduce in the oven, bake at 375 degrees F for 30 minutes and serve as a party dip.

Nutrition:

calories 186, fat 12.4, fiber 0.9, carbs 2.6, protein 1.5

Shrimp and Cucumber Bites

Prep Time: 5 min   **Cooking Time:** 0 min   **Servings:** 8

Ingredients:

- 1 big cucumber, cubed
- 1 pound shrimp, cooked, peeled, deveined and chopped 2 tablespoons heavy cream
- Salt and black pepper to the taste 12 whole grain crackers

Directions:

1. In a bowl, mix the cucumber with the rest of the ingredients except the crackers and stir well.

2. Arrange the crackers on a platter, spread the shrimp mix on each and serve.

Nutrition:

calories 155, fat 8.5, fiber 4.8, carbs 11.8, protein 17.7

Chili Mango and Watermelon Salsa

Prep Time: 5 min   **Cooking Time:** 0 min   **Servings:** 12

Ingredients:

- 1 red tomato, chopped
- Salt and black pepper to the taste
- cup watermelon, seedless, peeled and cubed 1 red onion, chopped
- mangos, peeled and chopped 2 chili peppers, chopped
- ¼ cup cilantro, chopped 3 tablespoons lime juice Pita chips for serving

Directions:

1. In a bowl, mix the tomato with the watermelon, the onion and the rest of the ingredients except the pita chips and toss well.
2. Divide the mix into small cups and serve with pita chips on the side.

Nutrition:

calories 62, fat 4.7, fiber 1.3, carbs 3.9, protein 2.3

Wrapped Plums

Prep Time: 5 min   **Cooking Time:** 0 min   **Servings:** 8

Ingredients:

- 2 ounces prosciutto, cut into 16 pieces 4 plums, quartered
- 1 tablespoon chives, chopped
- A pinch of red pepper flakes, crushed

Directions:

1. Wrap each plum quarter in a prosciutto slice, arrange them all on a platter, sprinkle the chives and pepper flakes all over and serve.

Nutrition:

calories 30, fat 1, fiber 0, carbs 4, protein 2

Zucchini and Olives Salsa

Prep Time: 5 min   **Cooking Time:** 0 min   **Servings:** 4

Ingredients:

- ½ cup black olives, pitted and sliced 3 zucchinis, cut with a spiralizer
- 1 cup cherry tomatoes, halved Salt and black pepper to the taste 1 small red onion, chopped
- ½ cup feta cheese, crumbled
- ½ cup olive oil
- ¼ cup apple cider vinegar

Directions:

1. In a bowl, mix the olives with the zucchinis and the rest of the ingredients, toss, divide into small cups and serve as an appetizer.

Nutrition:

calories 140, fat 14.2, fiber 1.4, carbs 3.5, protein 1.4

Salmon Rolls

Prep Time: 5 min   **Cooking Time:** 0 min   **Servings:** 12

Ingredients:

- 1 big long cucumber, thinly sliced lengthwise 2 teaspoons lime juice
- 4 ounces cream cheese, soft
- 1 teaspoon lemon zest, grated Salt and black pepper to the taste 2 teaspoons dill, chopped
- 4 ounces smoked salmon, cut into strips

Directions:

1. Arrange cucumber slices on a working surface and top each with a salmon strip.
2. In a bowl, mix the rest of the ingredients, stir and spread over the salmon.
3. Roll the salmon and cucumber strips, arrange them on a platter and serve as an appetizer.

Nutrition:

calories 245, fat 15.5, fiber 4.8, carbs 16.8, protein 17.3

Tomato Bruschetta

Prep Time: 10 min **Cooking Time:** 10 min **Servings:** 6

Ingredients:

- baguette, sliced
- 1/3 cup basil, chopped 6 tomatoes, cubed
- garlic cloves, minced
- A pinch of salt and black pepper 1 teaspoon olive oil
- 1 tablespoon balsamic vinegar
- ½ teaspoon garlic powder Cooking spray

Directions:

1. Arrange the baguette slices on a baking sheet lined with parchment paper, grease them with cooking spray and bake at 400 degrees F for 10 minutes.

2. In a bowl, mix the tomatoes with the basil and the remaining ingredients, toss well and leave aside for 10 minutes.

3. Divide the tomato mix on each baguette slice, arrange them all on a platter and serve.

Nutrition:

calories 162, fat 4 fiber 7, carbs 29, protein 4

Red Pepper Hummus

Prep Time: 10 min   **Cooking Time:** 0 min   **Servings:** 6

Ingredients:

- 6 ounces roasted red peppers, peeled and chopped 16 ounces canned chickpeas, drained and rinsed
- ¼ cup Greek yogurt
- 3 tablespoons tahini paste Juice of 1 lemon
- 3 garlic cloves, minced 1 tablespoon olive oil
- A pinch of salt and black pepper 1 tablespoon parsley, chopped

Directions:

1. In your food processor, combine the red peppers with the rest of the ingredients except the oil and the parsley and pulse well.

2. Add the oil, pulse again, divide into cups, sprinkle the parsley on top and serve as a party spread.

Nutrition:

calories 255, fat 11.4, fiber 4.5, carbs 17.4, protein 6.5

Olives and Cheese Stuffed Tomatoes

Prep Time: 10 min   **Cooking Time:** 0 min   **Servings:** 24

Ingredients:

- 24 cherry tomatoes, top cut off and insides scooped out 2 tablespoons olive oil
- ¼ teaspoon red pepper flakes
- ½ cup feta cheese, crumbled
- 2 tablespoons black olive paste
- ¼ cup mint, torn

Directions:

1. In a bowl, mix the olives paste with the rest of the ingredients except the cherry tomatoes and whisk well.

2. Stuff the cherry tomatoes with this mix, arrange them all on a platter and serve as an appetizer.

Nutrition:

calories 136, fat 8.6, fiber 4.8, carbs 5.6, protein 5.1

Goat Cheese and Chives Spread

Prep Time: 10 min   **Cooking Time:** 0 min   **Servings:** 4

Ingredients:

- 2 ounces goat cheese, crumbled
- ¾ cup sour cream
- 2 tablespoons chives, chopped 1 tablespoon lemon juice
- Salt and black pepper to the taste 2 tablespoons extra virgin olive oil

Directions:

1. In a bowl, mix the goat cheese with the cream and the rest of the ingredients and whisk really well.

2. Keep in the fridge for 10 minutes and serve as a party spread.

Nutrition:

calories 220, fat 11.5, fiber 4.8, carbs 8.9, protein 5.6

Lentils and Tomato Dip

Prep Time: 1 hour   **Cooking Tim:** 0 min   **Servings:** 6

Ingredients:

- 1 cup red lentils, cooked
- Salt and black pepper to the taste 2 tablespoons lemon juice
- garlic clove, minced
- tablespoons tomato paste
- 2 tablespoon cilantro, chopped 2 tablespoons olive oil
- 2 teaspoons cumin, ground

Directions:

1. In your blender, combine the lentils with the lemon juice, salt, pepper and the rest of the ingredients, and pulse well.

2. Transfer to a bowl and keep in the fridge for 1 hour before serving.

Nutrition:

calories 244, fat 8, fiber 12.4, carbs 26, protein 8.5

Lentils Spread

Prep Time: 2 hours   **Cooking Time:** 0 min   **Servings:** 12

Ingredients:

- 1 garlic clove, minced
- 12 ounces canned lentils, drained and rinsed 1 teaspoon oregano, dried
- ¼ teaspoon basil, dried 3 tablespoons olive oil
- tablespoon balsamic vinegar Salt and black pepper to the taste

Directions:

1. In a blender, combine the lentils with the garlic and the rest of the ingredients, pulse well, divide into bowls and serve as an appetizer.

Nutrition:

calories 287, fat 9.5, fiber 3.5, carbs 15.3, protein 9.3

Eggplant Bites

Prep Time: 10 min   **Cooking Time:** 15 min   **Servings:** 8

Ingredients:

- 2 eggplants, cut into 20 slices 2 tablespoons olive oil
- ½ cup roasted peppers, chopped
- ½ cup kalamata olives, pitted and chopped 1 tablespoon lime juice
- teaspoon red pepper flakes, crushed Salt and black pepper to the taste
- tablespoons mint, chopped

Directions:

1. In a bowl, mix the roasted peppers with the olives, half of the oil and the rest of the ingredients except the eggplant slices and stir well.

2. Brush eggplant slices with the rest of the olive oil on both sides, place them on the preheated grill over medium high heat, cook for 7 minutes on each side and transfer them to a platter.

3. Top each eggplant slice with roasted peppers mix and serve.

Nutrition:

calories 214, fat 10.6, fiber 5.8, carbs 15.4, protein 5.4

Walnuts Yogurt Dip

Prep Time: 5 min **Cooking Time:** 0 min **Servings:** 8

Ingredients:

- 3 garlic cloves, minced 2 cups Greek yogurt
- ¼ cup dill, chopped
- 1 tablespoon chives, chopped
- ¼ cup walnuts, chopped
- Salt and black pepper to the taste

Directions:

1. In a bowl, mix the garlic with the yogurt and the rest of the ingredients, whisk well, divide into small cups and serve as a party dip.

Nutrition:

calories 200, fat 6.5, fiber 4.6, carbs 15.5, protein 8.4, Fat 3.9 g, Carbohydrates 14.3 g, Sugar 7.3 g, Protein 2.5 g, Cholesterol 0 mg

Olive Eggplant Spread

Prep Time: 10 min   **Cooking Time:** 8 min   **Servings:** 12

Ingredients:

- 3/4 lbs eggplant, chopped 1/2 tbsp dried oregano
- 1/4 cup olives, pitted and chopped 1 tbsp tahini
- 1/4 cup fresh lime juice 1/2 cup water
- garlic cloves 1/4 cup olive oil Salt

Directions:

1. Add oil into the inner pot of instant pot and set the pot on sauté mode.
2. Add eggplant and cook for 3-5 minutes. Turn off sauté mode.
3. Add water and salt and stir well.
4. Seal pot with lid and cook on high for 3 minutes.
5. Once done, release pressure using quick release. Remove lid.
6. Drain eggplant well and transfer into the food processor.
7. Add remaining ingredients into the food processor and process until smooth.
8. Serve and enjoy.

Nutritional Value (Amount per Serving):

Calories 65, Fat 5.3 g, Carbohydrates 4.7 g, Sugar 2 g, Protein 0.9 g, Cholesterol 0 mg

Kidney Bean Spread

Prep Time: 10 min   **Cooking Time:** 18 min   **Servings:** 4

Ingredients:

- lb dry kidney beans, soaked overnight and drained 1 tsp garlic, minced
- tbsp olive oil
- 1 tbsp fresh lemon juice 1 tbsp paprika
- 4 cups vegetable stock 1/2 cup onion, chopped Pepper
- Salt

Directions:

1. Add beans and stock into the instant pot.
2. Seal pot with lid and cook on high for 18 minutes.
3. Once done, allow to release pressure naturally. Remove lid.
4. Drain beans well and reserve 1/2 cup stock.
5. Transfer beans, reserve stock, and remaining ingredients into the food processor and process until smooth.
6. Serve and enjoy.

Nutritional Value (Amount per Serving):

Calories 461, Fat 8.6 g, Carbohydrates 73 g, Sugar 4 g, Protein 26.4 g, Cholesterol 0 mg

Homemade Salsa

Prep Time: 10 min **Cooking Time:** 5 min **Servings:** 8

Ingredients:

- 12 oz grape tomatoes, halved 1/4 cup fresh cilantro, chopped 1 fresh lime juice
- 28 oz tomatoes, crushed 1 tbsp garlic, minced
- 1 green bell pepper, chopped
- 1 red bell pepper, chopped 2 onions, chopped
- 6 whole tomatoes Salt

Directions:

1. Add whole tomatoes into the instant pot and gently smash the tomatoes.
2. Add remaining ingredients except cilantro, lime juice, and salt and stir well.
3. Seal pot with lid and cook on high for 5 minutes.
4. Once done, allow to release pressure naturally for 10 minutes then release remaining using quick release. Remove lid.
5. Add cilantro, lime juice, and salt and stir well.
6. Serve and enjoy.

Nutritional Value (Amount per Serving):

Calories 146, Fat 1.2 g, Carbohydrates 33.2 g, Sugar 4 g, Protein 6.9 g, Cholesterol 0 mg

Healthy Spinach Dip

Prep Time: 10 min   **Cooking Time:** 8 min   **Servings:** 4

Ingredients:

- 14 oz spinach
- 2 tbsp fresh lime juice 1 tbsp garlic, minced 2 tbsp olive oil
- 2 tbsp coconut cream Pepper
- Salt

Directions:

1. Add all ingredients except coconut cream into the instant pot and stir well.
2. Seal pot with lid and cook on low pressure for 8 minutes.
3. Once done, allow to release pressure naturally for 5 minutes then release remaining using quick release. Remove lid.
4. Add coconut cream and stir well and blend spinach mixture using a blender until smooth.
5. Serve and enjoy.

Nutritional Value (Amount per Serving):

Calories 109, Fat 9.2 g, Carbohydrates 6.6 g, Sugar 1.1 g, Protein 3.2 g, Cholesterol 0 mg

Healthy Kidney Bean Dip

Prep Time: 10 min   **Cooking Time:** 10 min   **Servings:** 6

Ingredients:

- cup dry white kidney beans, soaked overnight and drained 1 tbsp fresh lemon juice
- tbsp water
- 1/2 cup coconut yogurt 1 roasted garlic clove 1 tbsp olive oil
- 1/4 tsp cayenne
- 1 tsp dried parsley Pepper
- Salt

Directions:

1. Add soaked beans and 1 3/4 cups of water into the instant pot.
2. Seal pot with lid and cook on high for 10 minutes.
3. Once done, allow to release pressure naturally. Remove lid.
4. Drain beans well and transfer them into the food processor.
5. Add remaining ingredients into the food processor and process until smooth.
6. Serve and enjoy.

Nutritional Value (Amount per Serving):

Calories 136, Fat 3.2 g, Carbohydrates 20 g, Sugar 2.1 g, Protein 7.7 g, Cholesterol 0 mg

Tomato Cucumber Salsa

Prep Time: 10 min   **Cooking Time:** 5 min   **Servings:** 4

Ingredients:

- 1 cucumber, chopped
- 1 1/2 lbs grape tomatoes, chopped 1 tbsp fresh chives, chopped
- tbsp fresh parsley, chopped 1 tbsp fresh basil, chopped
- onion, chopped 1/4 cup vinegar 2 tbsp olive oil
- 1/4 cup vegetable stock 2 chili peppers, chopped Pepper
- Salt

Directions:

1. Add tomatoes, stock, and chili peppers into the instant pot and stir well.
2. Seal pot with lid and cook on low pressure for 5 minutes.
3. Once done, allow to release pressure naturally for 5 minutes then release remaining using quick release. Remove lid.
4. Transfer tomato mixture into the mixing bowl.
5. Add remaining ingredients into the bowl and mix well.
6. Serve and enjoy.

Nutritional Value (Amount per Serving):

Calories 129, Fat 7.5 g, Carbohydrates 15 g, Sugar 8.3 g, Protein 2.7 g, Cholesterol 0 mg

Chocolate Hummus

Prep Time: 10 min   **Cooking Time:** 25 min   **Servings:** 10

Ingredients:

- 3/4 cup dried chickpeas, soaked overnight and drained 1 tsp vanilla
- 1/2 cup unsweetened cocoa powder 1/4 cup maple syrup
- 1/4 cup peanut butter 2 1/2 cups water Pinch of salt

Directions:

1. Add water and chickpeas into the instant pot.
2. Seal pot with lid and cook on high for 25 minutes.
3. Once done, release pressure using quick release. Remove lid.
4. Drain chickpeas well and reserved half cup of chickpea liquid.
5. Transfer chickpeas, reserved liquid, and remaining ingredients into the food processor and process until smooth.
6. Serve and enjoy.

Nutritional Value (Amount per Serving):

Calories 124, Fat 4.8 g, Carbohydrates 18 g, Sugar 7 g, Protein 5.4 g, Cholesterol 0 mg

Balsamic Bell Pepper Salsa

Prep Time: 10 min   **Cooking Time:** 6 min   **Servings:** 2

Ingredients:

- red bell peppers, chopped and seeds removed 1 cup grape tomatoes, halved
- 1/2 tbsp cayenne
- 1 tbsp balsamic vinegar 2 cup vegetable broth 1/2 cup sour cream
- 1/2 tsp garlic powder 1/2 onion, chopped Salt

Directions:

1. Add all ingredients except cream into the instant pot and stir well.
2. Seal pot with lid and cook on high for 6 minutes.
3. Once done, release pressure using quick release. Remove lid.
4. Add sour cream and stir well.
5. Blend the salsa mixture using an immersion blender until smooth.
6. Serve and enjoy.

Nutritional Value (Amount per Serving):

Calories 235, Fat 14.2 g, Carbohydrates 19.8 g, Sugar 10.7 g, Protein 9.2 g, Cholesterol 25 mg

Spicy Chicken Dip

Prep Time: 10min **Cooking Time:** 15 min **Servings:** 10

Ingredients:

- 1 lb chicken breast, skinless and boneless 1/2 cup sour cream
- 8 oz cheddar cheese, shredded 1/2 cup chicken stock
- 2 jalapeno pepper, sliced 8 oz cream cheese Pepper
- Salt

Directions:

1. Add chicken, stock, jalapenos, and cream cheese into the instant pot.
2. Seal pot with lid and cook on high for 12 minutes.
3. Once done, release pressure using quick release. Remove lid.
4. Shred chicken using a fork.
5. Set pot on sauté mode. Add remaining ingredients and stir well and cook until cheese is melted.
6. Serve and enjoy.

Nutritional Value (Amount per Serving):

Calories 248, Fat 19 g Carbohydrates 1.6 g, Sugar 0.3 g ,Protein 17.4 g, Cholesterol 83 mg

Perfect Italian Potatoes

Prep Time: 10 min   **Cooking Time:** 7 min   **Servings:** 6

Ingredients:

- 2 lbs baby potatoes, clean and cut in half 3/4 cup vegetable broth
- 6 oz Italian dry dressing mix

Directions:

1. Add all ingredients into the inner pot of instant pot and stir well.
2. Seal pot with lid and cook on high for 7 minutes.
3. Once done, allow to release pressure naturally for 3 minutes then release remaining using quick release. Remove lid.
4. Stir well and serve.

Nutritional Value (Amount per Serving):

Calories 149, Fat 0.3 g, Carbohydrates 41.6 g, Sugar 11.4 g, Protein 4.5 g, Cholesterol 0 mg

Jalapeno Chickpea Hummus

Prep Time: 10 min   **Cooking Time:** 25 min   **Servings:** 4

Ingredients:

- 1 cup dry chickpeas, soaked overnight and drained 1 tsp ground cumin
- 1/4 cup jalapenos, diced 1/2 cup fresh cilantro
- tbsp tahini 1/2 cup olive oil Pepper
- Salt

Directions:

1. Add chickpeas into the instant pot and cover with vegetable stock.
2. Seal pot with lid and cook on high for 25 minutes.
3. Once done, allow to release pressure naturally. Remove lid.
4. Drain chickpeas well and transfer into the food processor along with remaining ingredients and process until smooth.
5. Serve and enjoy.

Nutritional Value (Amount per Serving):

Calories 425, Fat 30.4 g, Carbohydrates 31.8 g, Sugar 5.6 g, Protein 10.5 g, Cholesterol 0 mg

Perfect Black Bean Dip

Prep Time: 10 min   **Cooking Time:** 30 min   **Servings:** 24

Ingredients:

- 1/2 cup dry black beans, rinsed and drained 1/2 tsp ground coriander
- 1/2 tsp chili powder 1 tsp paprika
- tsp ground cumin 1 fresh lime juice
- 1 1/2 tbsp olive oil
- 1 3/4 cup chicken broth 14 oz can tomatoes, diced 2 jalapenos, chopped
- 1 tbsp garlic, minced 1 onion, diced
- 1/2 tsp salt

Directions:

1. Add all ingredients into the instant pot and stir everything well.
2. Seal pot with lid and cook on high for 30 minutes.
3. Once done, allow to release pressure naturally for 10 minutes then release remaining using quick release. Remove lid.
4. Blend bean mixture using an immersion blender until smooth.
5. Serve and enjoy.

Nutritional Value (Amount per Serving):

Calories 59 Fat 1.2 g, Carbohydrates 9.4 g, Sugar 1.1 g, Protein 3.3 g, Cholesterol 143 mg

Delicious Eggplant Caponata

Prep Time: 10 min   **Cooking Time:** 5 min   **Servings:** 8

Ingredients:

- 1 eggplant, cut into 1/2-inch chunks 1 lb tomatoes, diced
- 1/2 cup tomato puree 1/4 cup dates, chopped 2 tbsp vinegar
- 1/2 cup fresh parsley, chopped 2 celery stalks, chopped
- small onion, chopped
- zucchini, cut into 1/2-inch chunks Pepper
- Salt

Directions:

1. Add all ingredients into the inner pot of instant pot and stir well.
2. Seal pot with lid and cook on high for 5 minutes.
3. Once done, release pressure using quick release. Remove lid.
4. Stir well and serve.

Nutritional Value (Amount per Serving):

Calories 60, Fat 0.4 g, Carbohydrates 14 g, Sugar 8.8 g, Protein 2.3 g, Cholesterol 0.4 mg

Tomato Olive Salsa

Prep Time: 10 min   **Cooking Time:** 5 min   **Servings:** 4

Ingredients:

- cups olives, pitted and chopped 1/4 cup fresh parsley, chopped 1/4 cup fresh basil, chopped
- 2 tbsp green onion, chopped 1 cup grape tomatoes, halved 1 tbsp olive oil
- tbsp vinegar Pepper
- Salt

Directions:

1. Add all ingredients into the inner pot of instant pot and stir well.
2. Seal pot with lid and cook on high for 5 minutes.
3. Once done, allow to release pressure naturally for 5 minutes then release remaining using quick release. Remove lid.
4. Stir well and serve.

Nutritional Value (Amount per Serving):

Calories 119, Fat 10.8 g, Carbohydrates 6.5 g, Sugar 1.3 g, Protein 1.2 g, Cholesterol 0 mg

Pepper Tomato Eggplant Spread

Prep Time: 10 min   **Cooking Time:** 10 min   **Servings:** 3

Ingredients:

- 2 cups eggplant, chopped 1/4 cup vegetable broth
- 2 tbsp tomato paste
- 1/4 cup sun-dried tomatoes, minced 1 cup bell pepper, chopped
- tsp garlic, minced 1 cup onion, chopped 3 tbsp olive oil
- Salt

Directions:

1. Add oil into the inner pot of instant pot and set the pot on sauté mode.
2. Add onion and sauté for 3 minutes.
3. Add eggplant, bell pepper, and garlic and sauté for 2 minutes.
4. Add remaining ingredients and stir well.
5. Seal pot with lid and cook on high for 5 minutes.
6. Once done, release pressure using quick release. Remove lid.
7. Lightly mash the eggplant mixture using a potato masher.
8. Stir well and serve.

Nutritional Value (Amount per Serving):

Calories 178, Fat 14.4 g, Carbohydrates 12.8 g, Sugar 7 g, Protein 2.4 g, Cholesterol 0 mg

Spicy Berry Dip

Prep Time: 10 min   **Cooking Time:** 15 min   **Servings:** 4

Ingredients:

- 10 oz cranberries
- 1/4 cup fresh orange juice 3/4 tsp paprika
- 1/2 tsp chili powder 1 tsp lemon zest
- 1 tbsp lemon juice

Directions:

1. Add all ingredients into the inner pot of instant pot and stir well.
2. Seal pot with lid and cook on high for 15 minutes.
3. Once done, allow to release pressure naturally for 5 minutes then release remaining using quick release. Remove lid.
4. Blend cranberry mixture using a blender until getting the desired consistency.
5. Serve and enjoy.

Nutritional Value (Amount per Serving):

Calories 49, Fat 0.2 g, Carbohydrates 8.6 g, Sugar 4.1 g, Protein 0.3 g, Cholesterol 0 mg

Parmesan Potatoes

Prep Time: 10 min   **Cooking Time:** 6 min   **Servings:** 4

Ingredients:

- lb potatoes, rinsed and cut into chunks 2 tbsp parmesan cheese, grated
- 2 tbsp olive oil 1/2 tsp parsley
- 1/2 tsp Italian seasoning 1 tsp garlic, minced
- 1 cup vegetable broth 1/2 tsp salt

Directions:

1. Add all ingredients except cheese into the instant pot and stir well.
2. Seal pot with lid and cook on high for 6 minutes.
3. Once done, release pressure using quick release. Remove lid.
4. Add parmesan cheese and stir until cheese is melted.
5. Serve and enjoy.

Nutritional Value (Amount per Serving):

Calories 237, Fat 8.3 g, Carbohydrates 36.3 g, Sugar 2.8 g, Protein 5.9 g, Cholesterol 2 mg

Garlic Thyme Chicken Drumsticks

Prep Time: 10 min   **Cooking Time:** 18 min   **Servings:** 4

Ingredients:

- 8 chicken drumsticks, skin-on 2 tbsp balsamic vinegar
- 2/3 cup can tomatoes, diced 6 garlic cloves
- 1 tsp lemon zest, grated 1 tsp dried thyme
- 1/4 tsp red pepper flakes
- 1 1/2 onions, cut into wedges 1 tbsp olive oil
- Pepper Salt

Directions:

1. Add oil into the inner pot of instant pot and set the pot on sauté mode.
2. Add onion and 1/2 tsp salt and sauté for 2-3 minutes.
3. Add chicken, garlic, lemon zest, red pepper flakes, and thyme and mix well.
4. Add vinegar and tomatoes and stir well.
5. Seal pot with lid and cook on high for 15 minutes.
6. Once done, release pressure using quick release. Remove lid.
7. Stir well and serve.

Nutritional Value (Amount per Serving):

Calories 220, Fat 8.9 g, Carbohydrates 7.8 g, Sugar 3.2 g, Protein 26.4 g, Cholesterol 81 mg

Tasty Turkey Chili

Prep Time: 10 min   **Cooking Time:** 25 min   **Servings:** 4

Ingredients:

- 1 lb cooked turkey, shredded 2 cups chicken broth
- 1 tsp tomato paste
- 1 small onion, chopped 1 tbsp Italian seasoning 1 tsp garlic powder
- tbsp cumin, roasted 1 tbsp chili powder
- cups tomatoes, crushed 1 tsp garlic, minced
- 14 oz can red beans, drained 14 oz can chickpeas, drained 1/2 cup corn
- 2 carrots, peeled and chopped 1/2 cup celery, chopped
- 1/4 cup edamame 2 tbsp olive oil Pepper
- Salt

Directions:

1. Add all ingredients into the instant pot and stir everything well.
2. Seal pot with lid and cook on high for 15 minutes.
3. Once done, allow to release pressure naturally. Remove lid.
4. Set pot on sauté mode and cook for 5-10 minutes or until chili thicken.
5. Stir well and serve.

Nutritional Value (Amount per Serving):

Calories 593, Fat 18.1 g, Carbohydrates 56 g, Sugar 7.3 g, Protein 50.9 g, Cholesterol 88 mg

Moist & Tender Turkey Breast

Prep Time: 10 min **Cooking Time:** 25 min **Servings:** 8

Ingredients:

- 4 lbs turkey breast, bone-in 1 tsp Italian seasoning
- 2 tbsp olive oil
- 14 oz chicken broth
- 1 celery ribs, chopped
- 1 large onion, cut into wedges 3/4 lbs carrots, cut into pieces Pepper
- Salt

Directions:

1. Add carrots, celery, onion, and broth into the instant pot and stir well.
2. Coat turkey breast with oil and season with Italian seasoning, pepper, and salt and place on top of vegetables into the instant pot.
3. Seal pot with lid and cook on high for 25 minutes.
4. Once done, allow to release pressure naturally for 10 minutes then release remaining using quick
5. release. Remove lid.
6. Slice and serve.

Nutritional Value (Amount per Serving):

Calories 301, Fat 7.7 g, Carbohydrates 15.9 g, Sugar 11.1 g, Protein 40.3 g, Cholesterol 98 mg

Herb Garlic Chicken

Prep Time: 10 min   **Cooking Time:** 12 min   **Servings:** 8

Ingredients:

- 4 lbs chicken breasts, skinless and boneless 1 tbsp garlic powder
- 2 tbsp dried Italian herb mix 2 tbsp olive oil
- 1/4 cup chicken stock Pepper
- Salt

Directions:

1. Coat chicken with oil and season with dried herb, garlic powder, pepper, and salt.

2. Place chicken into the instant pot. Pour stock over the chicken.

3. Seal pot with a lid and select manual and set timer for 12 minutes.

4. Once done, allow to release pressure naturally for 5 minutes then release remaining using quick release. Remove lid.

5. Shred chicken using a fork and serve.

Nutritional Value (Amount per Serving):

Calories 502, Fat 20.8 g, Carbohydrates 7.8 g, Sugar 1 g, Protein 66.8 g, Cholesterol 202 mg

Easy Chicken Scampi

Prep Time: 10 min   **Cooking Time:** 25 min   **Servings:** 4

Ingredients:

- 3 chicken breasts, skinless, boneless, and sliced 1 tsp garlic, minced
- 1 tbsp Italian seasoning 2 cups chicken broth
- 1 bell pepper, sliced 1/2 onion, sliced Pepper
- Salt

Directions:

1. Add chicken into the instant pot and top with remaining ingredients.
2. Seal pot with lid and cook on high for 25 minutes.
3. Once done, release pressure using quick release. Remove lid.
4. Remove chicken from pot and shred using a fork. Return shredded chicken to the pot and stir well.
5. Serve over cooked whole grain pasta and top with cheese.

Nutritional Value (Amount per Serving):

Calories 254, Fat 9.9 g, Carbohydrates 4.6 g, Sugar 2.8 g, Protein 34.6 g, Cholesterol 100 mg

Moroccan Spiced Chicken

Prep Time: 10 min   **Cooking Time:** 20 min   **Servings:** 4

Ingredients:

- 1 lb chicken thighs, boneless and cut into chunks
- 1 cup can tomato, crushed 1/2 tsp red pepper flakes 1 tsp dried parsley
- 1/2 tsp coriander 1 tsp cumin
- 14 oz can chickpeas, drained and rinsed 2 tomatoes, chopped
- tbsp garlic, minced 1 onion, sliced
- red peppers, diced 1 tbsp olive oil Pepper
- Salt

Directions:

1. Add oil into the inner pot of instant pot and set the pot on sauté mode.
2. Add onion and garlic and sauté for 5 minutes.
3. Add chicken and cook for 5 minutes.
4. Add remaining ingredients and stir well.
5. Seal pot with lid and cook on high for 10 minutes.
6. Once done, release pressure using quick release. Remove lid.
7. Stir well and serve.

Nutritional Value (Amount per Serving):

Calories 416 Fat 21.3 g, Carbohydrates 32.3 g, Sugar 4 g, Protein 26.1 g, Cholesterol 96 mg

Delicious Chicken Cacciatore

Prep Time: 10 min   **Cooking Time:** 18 min   **Servings:** 6

Ingredients:

- 6 chicken thighs, skinless and boneless 1 tbsp fresh parsley, chopped
- 1 tbsp fresh basil, chopped 1/4 cup olives, pitted
- 1/2 tsp dried oregano 1/4 tsp dried thyme
- 1 1/2 tbsp garlic, minced 1 carrot, sliced
- 1 bell pepper, chopped 2 tbsp tomato paste
- 28 oz fire-roasted tomatoes, crushed
- 1/2 onion, chopped 1 tbsp olive oil Pepper
- Salt

Directions:

1. Add oil into the inner pot of instant pot and set the pot on sauté mode.
2. Add onion and sauté for 3 minutes.
3. Add chicken and sauté for 3-5 minutes.
4. Add remaining ingredients except for olives, parsley, and basil and stir well.
5. Seal pot with lid and cook on high for 10 minutes.
6. Once done, allow to release pressure naturally. Remove lid.
7. Add olives, parsley, and basil and stir well.
8. Serve and enjoy.

Nutritional Value (Amount per Serving):

Calories 375, Fat 13.9 g, Carbohydrates 15.2 g, Sugar 8.4 g, Protein 43.1 g, Cholesterol 130 mg

Lemon Olive Chicken

Prep Time: 10 min   **Cooking Time:** 11 min   **Servings:** 8

Ingredients:

- lbs chicken breasts, skinless and boneless 4 oz olives, pitted
- 2 lemons, quartered and remove seeds
- 1 cinnamon stick
- 1 tsp turmeric powder 1 tsp ground coriander 1 tsp ground ginger
- tsp ground cumin 1 1/2 tsp paprika
- 1/2 cup chicken broth 1 tbsp garlic, minced 1 tbsp olive oil
- onions, sliced Pepper
- Salt

Directions:

1. Add chicken, lemon, cinnamon, turmeric, coriander, ginger, cumin, paprika, pepper, and salt into the zip-lock bag. Seal bag shake well and place in refrigerator overnight.

2. Add oil into the inner pot of instant pot and set the pot on sauté mode.

3. Add garlic and onion and sauté for 5 minutes.

4. Add marinated chicken, broth, and olives and stir well.

5. Seal pot with lid and cook on high for 6 minutes.

6. Once done, allow to release pressure naturally for 10 minutes then release remaining using quick release. Remove lid.

7. Stir and serve.

Nutritional Value (Amount per Serving):

Calories 271, Fat 12 g, Carbohydrates 6.1 g, Sugar 1.7 g, Protein 33.9 g, Cholesterol 101 mg

Protein Packed Chicken Bean Rice

Prep Time: 10 min   **Cooking Time:** 15 min   **Servings:** 6

Ingredients:

- 1 lb chicken breasts, skinless, boneless, and cut into chunks 14 oz can cannellini beans, rinsed and drained
- 4 cups chicken broth 2 cups brown rice
- 1 tbsp Italian seasoning 1 small onion, chopped 1 tbsp garlic, chopped 1 tbsp olive oil
- Pepper Salt

Directions:

1. Add oil into the inner pot of instant pot and set the pot on sauté mode.
2. Add garlic and onion and sauté for 3 minutes.
3. Add remaining ingredients and stir everything well.
4. Seal pot with a lid and select manual and set timer for 12 minutes.
5. Once done, release pressure using quick release. Remove lid.
6. Stir well and serve.

Nutritional Value (Amount per Serving):

Calories 494, Fat 11.3 g, Carbohydrates 61.4 g, Sugar 1.7 g, Protein 34.2 g, Cholesterol 69 mg

Creamy Chicken Breasts

Prep Time: 10 min   **Cooking Time:** 12 min   **Servings:** 4

Ingredients:

- 4 chicken breasts, skinless and boneless 1 tbsp basil pesto
- 1 1/2 tbsp cornstarch
- 1/4 cup roasted red peppers, chopped 1/3 cup heavy cream
- 1 tsp Italian seasoning 1 tsp garlic, minced
- cup chicken broth Pepper
- Salt

Directions:

1. Add chicken into the instant pot. Season chicken with Italian seasoning, pepper, and salt. Sprinkle with garlic.

2. Pour broth over chicken. Seal pot with lid and cook on high for 8 minutes.

3. Once done, allow to release pressure naturally for 5 minutes then release remaining using quick release. Remove lid.

4. Transfer chicken on a plate and clean the instant pot.

5. Set instant pot on sauté mode. Add heavy cream, pesto, cornstarch, and red pepper to the pot and stir well and cook for 3-4 minutes.

6. Return chicken to the pot and coat well with the sauce.

7. Serve and enjoy.

Nutritional Value (Amount per Serving):

Calories 341, Fat 15.2 g, Carbohydrates 4.4 g, Sugar 0.8 g, Protein 43.8 g, Cholesterol 144 mg

Pesto Vegetable Chicken

Prep Time: 10 min   **Cooking Time:** 25 min   **Servings:** 4

Ingredients:

- 1 1/2 lbs chicken thighs, skinless, boneless, and cut into pieces 1/2 cup chicken broth
- 1/4 cup fresh parsley, chopped 2 cups cherry tomatoes, halved 1 cup basil pesto
- 3/4 lb asparagus, trimmed and cut in half
- 2/3 cup sun-dried tomatoes, drained and chopped 2 tbsp olive oil
- Pepper
- Salt

Directions:

1. Add oil into the inner pot of instant pot and set the pot on sauté mode.
2. Add chicken and sauté for 5 minutes.
3. Add remaining ingredients except for tomatoes and stir well.
4. Seal pot with a lid and select manual and set timer for 15 minutes.
5. Once done, release pressure using quick release. Remove lid.
6. Add tomatoes and stir well. Again seal the pot and select manual and set timer for 5 minutes.
7. Release pressure using quick release. Remove lid.
8. Stir well and serve.

Nutritional Value (Amount per Serving):

Calories 459, Fat 20.5 g, Carbohydrates 14.9 g, Sugar 9.2 g, Protein 9.2 g, Cholesterol 151 mg

Zesty Veggie Chicken

Prep Time: 10 min   **Cooking Time:** 5 min   **Servings:** 4

Ingredients:

- 1 lb chicken tender, skinless, boneless and cut into chunks 10 oz of frozen vegetables
- 1/3 cup zesty Italian dressing 1/2 tsp Italian seasoning
- 1 cup fried onions 2/3 cup rice
- 1 cup chicken broth Pepper
- Salt

Directions:

1. Add all ingredients except vegetables into the instant pot.

2. Meanwhile, cook frozen vegetables in microwave according to packet instructions.

3. Seal pot with lid and cook on high for 5 minutes.

4. Once done, allow to release pressure naturally for 10 minutes then release remaining using quick release. Remove lid.

5. Add cooked vegetables and stir well.

6. Serve and enjoy.

Nutritional Value (Amount per Serving):

Calories 482, Fat 15.9 g, Carbohydrates 40.5 g, Sugar 2.6 g, Protein 38.3 g, Cholesterol 101 mg

Quick Chicken with Mushrooms

Prep Time: 10 min   **Cooking Time:** 22 min   **Servings:** 6

Ingredients:

- lbs chicken breasts, skinless and boneless 1/2 cup heavy cream
- 1/3 cup water
- 3/4 lb mushrooms, sliced 3 tbsp olive oil
- 1 tsp Italian seasoning Pepper
- Salt

Directions:

1. Add oil into the inner pot of instant pot and set the pot on sauté mode.
2. Season chicken with Italian seasoning, pepper, and salt.
3. Add chicken to the pot and sauté for 5 minutes. Remove chicken from pot and set aside.
4. Add mushrooms and sauté for 5 minutes or until mushrooms are lightly brown.
5. Return chicken to the pot. Add water and stir well.
6. Seal pot with a lid and select manual and set timer for 12 minutes.
7. Once done, release pressure using quick release. Remove lid.
8. Remove chicken from pot and place on a plate.
9. Set pot on sauté mode. Add heavy cream and stir well and cook for 5 minutes.
10. Pour mushroom sauce over chicken and serve.

Nutritional Value (Amount per Serving):

Calories 396, Fat 22.3 g, Carbohydrates 2.2 g, Sugar 1.1 g, Protein 45.7 g, Cholesterol 149 mg

Greek Chicken Rice

Prep Time: 10 min   **Cooking Time:** 14 min   **Servings:** 4

Ingredients:

- 3 chicken breasts, skinless, boneless, and cut into chunks 1/4 fresh parsley, chopped
- zucchini, sliced
- bell peppers, chopped
- 1 cup rice, rinsed and drained 1 1/2 cup chicken broth
- 1 tbsp oregano
- 3 tbsp fresh lemon juice 1 tbsp garlic, minced
- onion, diced 2 tbsp olive oil Pepper
- Salt

Directions:

1. Add oil into the inner pot of instant pot and set the pot on sauté mode.
2. Add onion and chicken and cook for 5 minutes.
3. Add rice, oregano, lemon juice, garlic, broth, pepper, and salt and stir everything well.
4. Seal pot with lid and cook on high for 4 minutes.
5. Once done, release pressure using quick release. Remove lid.
6. Add parsley, zucchini, and bell peppers and stir well.
7. Seal pot again with lid and select manual and set timer for 5 minutes.
8. Release pressure using quick release. Remove lid.
9. Stir well and serve.

Nutritional Value (Amount per Serving):

Calories 500 Fat 16.5 g, Carbohydrates 48 g, Sugar 5.7 g, Protein 38.7 g, Cholesterol 97 mg

Perfect Chicken & Rice

Prep Time: 10 min   **Cooking Time:** 25 min   **Servings:** 4

Ingredients:

- 1 lb chicken breasts, skinless and boneless 1 tsp olive oil
- 1 cup onion, diced 1 tsp garlic minced
- 4 carrots, peeled and sliced
- tbsp Mediterranean spice mix 2 cups brown rice, rinsed
- cups chicken stock Pepper
- Salt

Directions:

1. Add oil into the inner pot of instant pot and set the pot on sauté mode.
2. Add garlic and onion and sauté until onion is softened.
3. Add stock, carrot, rice, and Mediterranean spice mix and stir well.
4. Place chicken on top of rice mixture and season with pepper and salt. Do not mix.
5. Seal pot with a lid and select manual and set timer for 20 minutes.
6. Once done, allow to release pressure naturally for 10 minutes then release remaining using quick release. Remove lid.
7. Remove chicken from pot and shred using a fork.
8. Return shredded chicken to the pot and stir well.
9. Serve and enjoy.

Nutritional Value (Amount per Serving):

Calories 612, Fat 12.4 g, Carbohydrates 81.7 g, Sugar 4.6 g, Protein 41.1 g, Cholesterol 101 mg

Chicken and Artichokes

Prep Time: 10 min   **Cooking Time:** 20 min   **Servings:** 4

Ingredients:

- 2 pounds chicken breast, skinless, boneless and sliced A pinch of salt and black pepper
- 4 tablespoons olive oil
- 8 ounces canned roasted artichoke hearts, drained 6 ounces sun-dried tomatoes, chopped
- 3 tablespoons capers, drained 2 tablespoons lemon juice

Directions:

1. Heat up a pan with half of the oil over medium-high heat, add the artichokes and the other ingredients except the chicken, stir and sauté for 10 minutes.

2. Transfer the mix to a bowl, heat up the pan again with the rest of the oil over medium-high heat, add the meat and cook for 4 minutes on each side.

3. Return the veggie mix to the pan, toss, cook everything for 2-3 minutes more, divide between plates and serve.

Nutrition:

calories 552, fat 28, fiber 6, carbs 33, protein 43

Paprika Chicken and Pineapple Mix

Prep Time: 10 min   **Cooking Time:** 15 min   **Servings:** 4

Ingredients:

- 2 cups pineapple, peeled and cubed
- 2 tablespoons olive oil
- 1tablespoon smoked paprika
- 2pounds chicken breasts, skinless, boneless and cubed A pinch of salt and black pepper
- 1 tablespoon chives, chopped

Directions:

1. Heat up a pan with the oil over medium-high heat, add the chicken, salt and pepper and brown for 4 minutes on each side.
2. Add the rest of the ingredients, toss, cook for 7 minutes more, divide everything between plates and serve with a side salad.

Nutrition:

calories 264, fat 13.2, fiber 8.3, carbs 25.1, protein 15.4

Brown Rice, Chicken and Scallions

Prep Time: 10 min   **Cooking Time:** 30 min   **Servings:** 4

Ingredients:

- 1and ½ cups brown rice 3 cups chicken stock
- 2tablespoon balsamic vinegar
- 1pound chicken breast, boneless, skinless and cubed 6 scallions, chopped
- Salt and black pepper to the taste 1 tablespoon sweet paprika
- 2tablespoons avocado oil

Directions:

1. Heat up a pan with the oil over medium-high heat, add the chicken and brown for 5 minutes.

2. Add the scallions and sauté for 5 minutes more.

3. Add the rice and the rest of the ingredients, bring to a simmer and cook over medium heat for 20 minutes.

4. Stir the mix, divide everything between plates and serve.

Nutrition:

calories 300, fat 9.2, fiber 11.8, carbs 18.6, protein 23.8

CONCLUSION

Thank you for reaching the end of this book, "Mediterranean Diet Cookbook for Beginners". I hope you enjoyed reading it as much as I had while writing it. As you can now see, the Mediterranean diet is not a restrictive one and it's so easy to follow. As you can also see, it's all about living a healthy and happy life – it's not about being skinny or losing weight – it's about how to adjust your diet to make you healthier and happier.

In comparison to other diets out there, Mediterranean Diet is low in saturated fat, cholesterol, trans-fat and sodium. It also lows in total fat, polyunsaturated fat, and has a moderate amount of carbohydrates. So even though Mediterranean Diet is low in total fat, it has a moderate amount of saturated fat and a nice amount of monounsaturated fats. It is extremely high in dietary fiber, which means you get all the fiber you need with this diet.

The Mediterranean diet actually is more positively defined by dietary patterns than by single food items. The diet emphasizes eating primarily plant-derived foods with olive oil. However, this diet doesn't prescribe that you must eat a particular food.

The Mediterranean diet emphasizes getting more vegetables, fruits, grains, beans, seeds, nuts, legumes, herbs, and spices. It also stresses eating fish and seafood (no red meat usually) and poultry, as well as using wine in moderation. It is all about balance and moderation, and it's about eating fresh, unprocessed foods, plenty of fruits and vegetables, whole grains, beans, seeds, nuts, legumes, herbs and spices. It is about being active every day and not eating too much.

The Mediterranean diet avoids processed foods preferring to use fresh foods. You can eat so many wonderful and delicious dishes from the Mediterranean diet, and now you can have all the recipes you need in "Mediterranean Diet Cookbook for Beginners" to help change your lifestyle for the better.

Here are some tips for you to continually maintain this diet:

1. Balance your diet
2. Eat more frequently, but in smaller portions
3. Don't skip meals
4. Maintain a healthy consistency in your meals
5. Give it time to adjust your body to the new foods and ingredients
6. Make the change realistic and achievable
7. Eliminate processed and refined foods from your diet
8. Don't be afraid of eating a variety of foods
9. Don't deprive yourself of treats
10. Keep a food diary
11. Don't be too hard on yourself
12. Take a walk after meals
13. Go for a swim or do some more exercise
14. Stay positive. You're worth this diet and the new lifestyle it has to offer you.

I would like you to think about what you can do with the knowledge that you now have. The main thing is to go out and try the recipes. Cook them for your loved ones, or for friends and family. Cook and enjoy. You have no obligation to follow what I have written here.

The other best thing to do is try to cook Mediterranean dishes yourself – thinking about your diet changes and see how delicious the food can be.

The Mediterranean diet will change the way you look in a matter of days. It will improve your bowel movements and digestion in a matter of days. It will keep you fuller for longer. It will increase your energy and improve your mood. These things happen to everyone who tries this diet, if you follow it correctly. Thank you for reading my book, and I hope that it will help you change your life and that of your loved ones in a very positive way.

To your health and happiness.

Again, thank you for your time. So now you have a great way to start your healthy Mediterranean lifestyle.

CPSIA information can be obtained
at www.ICGtesting.com
Printed in the USA
BVHW050042080421
604338BV00008BA/892